Dash Diet Cookbook

A Complete Dash Diet Plan for Your Delicious Meals

Eleonore Barlow

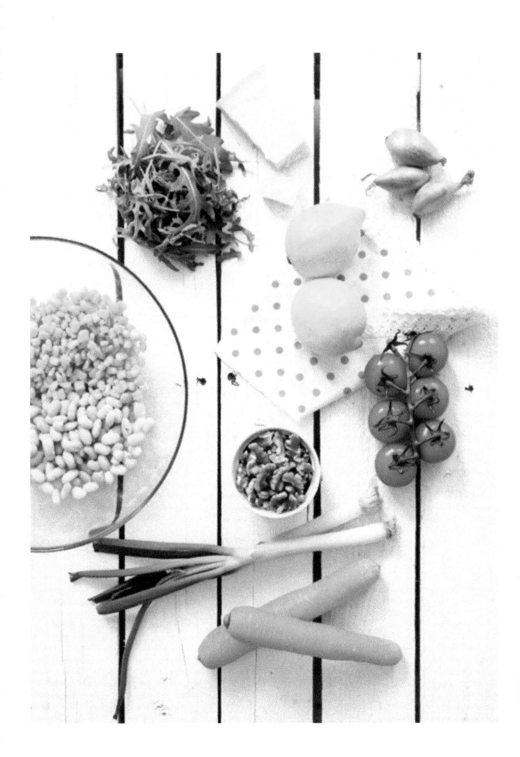

Table of Contents

Italian Turkey Sausage and Vegetable Omelet

You can prepare this hearty 20-minute entrée for breakfast, lunch, or dinner, and it is perfect for one-person cooking.

The omelet fills with chicken sausage, onion, mushrooms, and roasted red peppers, then finished with salty Pecorino Romano cheese, which is chopped parsley. This addition injects freshness and color. Italian sausages come in several varieties that are sweet and spicy, so use your favorite in this recipe. When preparing omelets, it's good to practice to cook all the fillings and get them ready to go before you start cooking the eggs, since the cooking process is a quick one that takes only a couple minutes per omelet.

SmartPoints value: Green plan - 6SP, Blue plan - 2SP, Purple plan - 2SP Total Time: 20 min, Prep time: 10 min, Cooking time: 10 min, Serves: 1 Nutritional value: Calories - 292.3, Carbs - 5.1g, Fat - 21.4g, Protein - 22.9g

Ingredients

Cooked chicken or turkey sausage(s) - 1½ oz, Italian-variety, chopped

Fresh edible mushroom(s) - ¾ cup(s), chopped

Fresh parsley - ½ Tbsp, chopped

Uncooked onion(s) - ¼ cup(s), chopped

Cooking spray - 4 spray(s)

Egg(s) - 2 large, beaten with a pinch of salt and pepper

Grated Pecorino Romano cheese - 1½ Tbsp

Chopped and roasted red peppers (packed in water) - ¼ cup(s)

Instructions

1.   Coat a small-sized omelet pan with cooking spray and heat over medium flame.

2.   Add the sausage, mushroom, and onion, then cook, frequently stirring, until the onions soften, 5 minutes. Remove the cooked omelet from pan to a bowl and stir in roasted pepper, then set aside.

3.   Wipe the pan clean with a paper towel.

4.   Put off heat, coat the pan again with cooking spray, and heat over medium flame.

5.   Add the beaten eggs and swirl to spread egg over the pan.

6.   Cook it until the bottom is done and the top is nearly cooked for about 3 minutes.

7.   Top the omelet with chicken sausage mixture and sprinkle with cheese.

8.   Fold the omelet over and cook for 1-2 minutes more. Serve it sprinkled with parsley.

Chinese-Style Zucchini with Ginger

Servings per container - 10

Prep Total - 10 min

Serving Size 2/3 cup (55g)

Nutritional Facts

Total Fat 8g

Total Carbohydrate 37g

Protein 3g

Sodium 160mg

Ingredients:

1 teaspoon oil

1 lb. zucchini cut into 1/4-inch slices

1/2 cup vegetarian broth

2 teaspoon light soy sauce

1 teaspoon dry sherry

1 teaspoon toasted sesame oil

Instructions:

1.   Heat a large wok or heavy skillets over high heat until very hot then add the oil. When the oil is hot, add the zucchini and ginger.

2.   Stir-fry 1 minute.

3.   Add the broth, soy sauce, and sherry.

4.   Stir-fry over high heat until the broth cooks down a bit and the zucchini is crisp-tender.

5.   Remove from the heat, sprinkle with sesame oil and serve.

Breakfast Super Antioxidant Berry Smoothie

servings per container - 5

Prep Total - 10 min

Serving Size - 4 cup (20g)

Nutritional Facts

Total Fat 2g

Sodium 7mg

Total Carbohydrate 20g

Protein 3g

Ingredients

1 cup of filtered water

1 whole orange, peeled, de-seeded & cut into chunks

2 cups frozen raspberries or blackberries

1 Tablespoon goji berries

1 1/2 Tablespoons hemp seeds or plant-based protein powder

2 cups leafy greens (parsley, spinach, or kale)

Instructions:

Blend on high until smooth

Serve and drink immediately

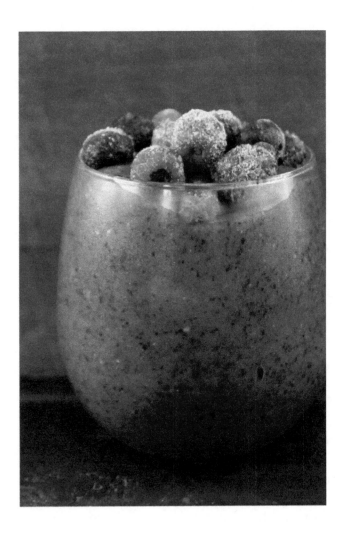

Cucumber Tomato Surprise

servings per container - 5

Prep Total - 10 min

Serving Size 2/3 cup (55g)

Nutritional Facts

Total Fat 20g

Total Carbohydrate 14g

Total Sugar 2g

Protein 7g

Ingredients

Chopped 1 medium of tomato

1 small cucumber peeled in stripes and chopped

1 large avocado cut into cubes

1 half of a lemon or lime squeezed

½21 tsp. Himalayan or Real salt

1 Teaspoon of original olive oil, MCT or coconut oil

Instructions:

1.   Mix everything together and enjoy

2.   This dish tastes even better after sitting for 40 – 60 minutes

3.   Blend into a soup if desired.

Avocado Nori Rolls

Nutritional Facts

servings per container	10
Prep Total	**10 min**
Serving Size 2/3 cup (70g)	
Amount per serving **Calories**	**15**
	% Daily Value
Total Fat 2g	**10%**
Saturated Fat 1g	9%
Trans Fat 10g	-
Cholesterol	**1%**
Sodium 70mg	**5%**
Total Carbohydrate 22g	**40%**
Dietary Fiber 4g	2%
Total Sugar 12g	-
Protein 3g	
Vitamin C 2mcg	2%
Calcium 260mg	7%
Iron 8mg	2%
Potassium 235mg	4%

Ingredients

2 sheets of raw or toasted sushi nori

1 large Romaine leaf cut in half down the length of the spine

2 Teaspoon of spicy miso paste

1 avocado, peeled and sliced

½ red, yellow or orange bell pepper, julienned

½ cucumber, peeled, seeded and julienned

½ cup raw sauerkraut

½ carrot, beet or zucchini, shredded

1 cup alfalfa or favorite green sprouts

1 small bowl of water for sealing roll

Instructions:

1. Place a sheet of nori on a sushi rolling mat or washcloth, lining it up at the end closest to you.

2. Place the Romaine leaf on the edge of the nori with the spine closest to you.

3. Spread Spicy Miso Paste on the Romaine

4. Line the leaf with all ingredients in descending order, placing sprouts on last

5. Roll the Nori sheet away from you, tucking the ingredients in with your fingers, and seal the roll with water or Spicy Miso Paste. Slice the roll into 6 or 8 rounds.

Maple Ginger Pancakes

Nutritional Facts

servings per container	4
Prep Total	**10 min**
Serving Size 2/3 cup (20g)	
Amount per serving **Calories**	**20**
	% Daily Value
Total Facts 10g	**10%**
Saturated Fat 0g	7%
Trans **Fat** 2g	-
Cholesterol	**3%**
Sodium 10mg	**2%**
Total Carbohydrate 7g	**3%**
Dietary Fiber 2g	4%
Total Sugar 1g	-
Protein 3g	
Vitamin C 2mcg	10%
Calcium 260mg	20%
Iron 8mg	30%
Potassium 235mg	6%

Ingredients

1 or 2 cup flour

1 tablespoonful baking powder

1/2 tablespoonful kosher salt

1/4 tablespoonful ground ginger

1/4 table spoonful pumpkin pie spice

1/3 cup maple syrup

2/4 cup water

minced 1/4 cup + 1 tablespoonful crystallized ginger slices together

Instructions:

1.   In a neat bowl mix together the first five recipes

2.   Add flour with syrup with water and stir together, after that add in the chopped ginger & stir until-just-combined.

3.   Heat your frying pan and coat with a nonstick cooking spray

4.   Pour in 1/4 cup of the batter and allow to heat until it forms bubbles. Allow to cook until browned

5.   Serve warm & topped with a slathering of vegan butter, a splash of maple syrup, and garnished with chopped candied ginger.

Chewy Chocolate Chip Cookies

Nutritional Facts

servings per container	10
Prep Total	**10 min**
Serving Size 2/3 cup (40g)	
Amount per serving **Calories**	**10**
	% Daily Value
Total Fat 10g	**2%**
Saturated Fat 1g	5%
Trans Fat 0g	-
Cholesterol	**15%**
Sodium 120mg	**8%**
Total Carbohydrate 21g	**10%**
Dietary Fiber 4g	1%
Total Sugar 1g	0%
Protein 6g	
Vitamin C 2mcg	7%
Calcium 210mg	51%
Iron 8mg	1%
Potassium 235mg	10%

Ingredients

1 cup vegan butter, softened

½ cup white sugar

½ cup brown sugar

¼ cup dairy-free milk

1 teaspoon vanilla

2 ¼ cups flour

½ teaspoon salt

1 teaspoon baking soda

12 ounces dairy-free chocolate chips

Instructions:

1.   Preheat oven to 350°F.

2.   In a large bowl, mix the butter, white sugar, and brown sugar until light and fluffy. Slowly stir in the dairy-free milk and then add the vanilla to make a creamy mixture.

3.   In a separate bowl, combine the flour, salt, and baking soda.

4.   You need to add this dry mixture to the liquid mixture and stir well. Fold in the chocolate chips.

5.   Drop small spoonful of the batter onto non-stick cookie sheets and bake for 9 minutes.

Lovely Faux Mac and Cheese

Serving: 4

Prep Time: 15 minutes

Cook Time: 45 minutes

Ingredients:

5 cups cauliflower florets

Sunflower seeds and pepper to taste

1 cup coconut almond milk

½ cup vegetable broth

2 tablespoons coconut flour, sifted

1 organic egg, beaten

1 cup cashew cheese

How To:

1.   Preheat your oven to 350 degrees F.

2.   Season florets with sunflower seeds and steam until firm.

3.   Place florets during a greased ovenproof dish.

4.   Heat coconut almond milk over medium heat during a skillet, confirm to season the oil with sunflower seeds and pepper.

5.   Stir in broth and add coconut flour to the combination, stir.

6.   Cook until the sauce begins to bubble.

7.   Remove heat and add beaten egg.

8.   Pour the thick sauce over the cauliflower and blend in cheese.

9.   Bake for 30-45 minutes.

10.   Serve and enjoy!

Nutrition (Per Serving)

Calories: 229

Fat: 14g

Carbohydrates: 9g

Protein: 15g

Epic Mango Chicken

Serving: 4

Prep Time: 25 minutes

Cook Time: 10 minutes

Ingredients:

2 medium mangoes, peeled and sliced

10-ounce coconut almond milk

4 teaspoons vegetable oil

4 teaspoons spicy curry paste

14-ounce chicken breast halves, skinless and boneless, cut in cubes

4 medium shallots

1 large English cucumber, sliced and seeded

How To:

1.   Slice half the mangoes and add the halves to a bowl.

2.   Add mangoes and coconut almond milk to a blender and blend until you've got a smooth puree.

23

3.   Keep the mixture on the side.

4.   Take a large-sized pot and place it over medium heat, add oil and permit the oil to heat up.

5.   Add curry paste and cook for 1 minute until you've got a pleasant fragrance, add shallots and chicken to the pot and cook for five minutes.

6.   Pour mango puree in to the combination and permit it to heat up.

7.   Serve the cooked chicken with mango puree and cucumbers.

8.   Enjoy!

Nutrition (Per Serving)

Calories: 398

Fat: 20g

Carbohydrates: 32g

Protein: 26g

Chicken and Cabbage Platter

Serving: 2

Prep Time: 9 minutes

Cook Time: 14 minutes

Ingredients:

½ cup sliced onion

1 tablespoon sesame garlic-flavored oil 2cups shredded Bok-Choy 1/2 cups fresh bean sprouts

1 1/2 stalks celery, chopped

1 ½ teaspoons minced garlic

1/2 teaspoon stevia

1/2 cup chicken broth

1 tablespoon coconut aminos

1/2 tablespoon freshly minced ginger

1/2 teaspoon arrowroot

2 boneless chicken breasts, cooked and sliced thinly

How To:

1.   Shred the cabbage with a knife.

2.   Slice onion and increase your platter alongside the rotisserie chicken.

3.   Add a dollop of mayonnaise on top and drizzle vegetable oil over the cabbage.

4.   Season with sunflower seeds and pepper consistent with your taste.

5.   Enjoy!

Nutrition (Per Serving)

Calories: 368

Fat: 18g

Net Carbohydrates: 8g

Protein: 42g

Fiber: 3g

Carbohydrates: 11g

Hearty Chicken Liver Stew

Serving: 2

Prep Time: 10 minutes

Cook Time: Nil

Ingredients:

10 ounces chicken livers

1-ounce onion, chopped

2 ounces sour cream

1 tablespoon olive oil

Sunflower seeds to taste

How To:

1.   Take a pan and place it over medium heat.

2.   Add oil and let it heat up.

3.   Add onions and fry until just browned.

4.   Add livers and season with sunflower seeds.

5.   Cook until livers are half cooked.

6.   Transfer the combination to a stew pot.

7.   Add soured cream and cook for 20 minutes.

8.   Serve and enjoy!

Nutrition (Per Serving)

Calories: 146

Fat: 9g

Carbohydrates: 2g

Protein: 15g

Chicken Quesadilla

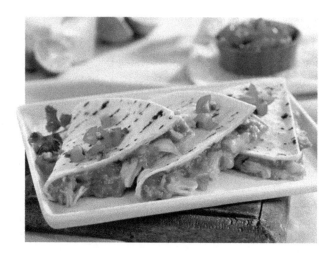

Serving: 2

Prep Time: 10 minutes

Cook Time: 35 minutes

Ingredients:

¼ cup ranch dressing

½ cup cheddar cheese, shredded

20 slices bacon, center-cut

2 cups grilled chicken, sliced

How To:

1. Re-heat your oven to 400 degrees F.

2. Line baking sheet using parchment paper.

3. Weave bacon into two rectangles and bake for half-hour.

4. Lay grilled chicken over bacon square, drizzling ranch dressing on top.

5. Sprinkle cheddar and top with another bacon square.

6. Bake for five minutes more.

7. Slice and serve.

8. Enjoy!

Nutrition (Per Serving)

Calories: 619

Fat: 35g

Carbohydrates: 2g

Protein: 79g

Zucchini Beef Sauté with Coriander Greens

Serving: 4

Prep Time: 10 minutes

Cook Time: 10 minutes

Ingredients:

10 ounces beef, sliced into 1-2-inch strips

1 zucchini, cut into 2-inch strips

¼ cup parsley, chopped

3 garlic cloves, minced

2 tablespoons tamari sauce

4 tablespoons avocado oil

How To:

1.   Add 2 tablespoons avocado oil during a frypan over high heat.

2.   Place strips of beef and brown for a couple of minutes on high heat.

3.   Once the meat is brown, add zucchini strips and sauté until tender.

4.   Once tender, add tamari sauce, garlic, parsley and allow them to sit for a couple of minutes more.

5.   Serve immediately and enjoy!

Nutrition (Per Serving)

Calories: 500

Fat: 40g

Carbohydrates: 5g

Protein: 31g

Hearty Lemon and Pepper Chicken

Serving: 4

Prep Time: 5 minutes

Cook Time: 15

Ingredients:

2 teaspoons olive oil

1 ¼ pounds skinless chicken cutlets

2 whole eggs

¼ cup panko crumbs

1 tablespoon lemon pepper

Sunflower seeds and pepper to taste

3 cups green beans

¼ cup parmesan cheese

¼ teaspoon garlic powder

How To:

1.   Pre-heat your oven to 425 degrees F.

2.   Take a bowl and stir in seasoning, parmesan, lemon pepper, garlic powder, panko.

3.   Whisk eggs in another bowl.

4.   Coat cutlets in eggs and press into panko mix.

5.   Transfer coated chicken to a parchment lined baking sheet.

6.   Toss the beans in oil, pepper, add sunflower seeds, and lay them on the side of the baking sheet.

7.   Bake for quarter-hour.

8.   Enjoy!

Nutrition (Per Serving)

Calorie: 299

Fat: 10g

Carbohydrates: 10g

Protein: 43g

Walnuts and Asparagus Delight

Serving: 4

Prep Time: 5 minutes

Cook Time: 5 minutes

Ingredients:

1 ½ tablespoons olive oil

¾ pound asparagus, trimmed

¼ cup walnuts, chopped

Sunflower seeds and pepper to taste

How To:

1.   Place a skillet over medium heat add vegetable oil and let it heat up.

2.   Add asparagus, sauté for five minutes until browned.

3.   Season with sunflower seeds and pepper.

4.   Remove heat.

5.   Add walnuts and toss.

6.   Serve warm!

Nutrition (Per Serving)

Calories: 124

Fat: 12g

Carbohydrates: 2g

Protein: 3g

Healthy Carrot Chips

Serving: 4

Prep Time: 10 minutes

Cook Time: 10 minutes

Ingredients:

3 cups carrots, sliced paper-thin rounds

2 tablespoons olive oil

2 teaspoons ground cumin

½ teaspoon smoked paprika Pinch of sunflower seeds

How To:

1.   Pre-heat your oven to 400 degrees F.

2.   Slice carrot into thin shaped coins employing a peeler.

3.   Place slices during a bowl and toss with oil and spices.

4.   Lay out the slices on a parchment paper, lined baking sheet during a single layer.

5.   Sprinkle sunflower seeds.

6.   Transfer to oven and bake for 8-10 minutes.

7.   Remove and serve.

Enjoy!

Nutrition (Per Serving)

Calories: 434

Fat: 35g

Carbohydrates: 31g

Protein: 2g

Garden Vegetable and Herb Soup

Total Time

Prep: 20 min. Cook: 30 min.

Makes

8 servings (2 quarts)

Ingredients:

2 tablespoons olive oil

2 medium onions, hacked

2 huge carrots, cut

1 pound red potatoes (around 3 medium), cubed

2 cups of water

1 can (14-1/2 ounces) diced tomatoes in sauce

1-1/2 cups vegetable soup

1-1/2 teaspoons garlic powder

1 teaspoon dried basil

1/2 teaspoon salt

1/2 teaspoon paprika

1/4 teaspoon dill weed

1/4 teaspoon pepper

1 medium yellow summer squash, split and cut

1 medium zucchini, split and cut

Directions:

1. In a huge pan, heat oil over medium warmth. Include onions and carrots; cook and mix until onions are delicate, 4-6 minutes. Include potatoes and cook 2 minutes. Mix in water, tomatoes, juices, and seasonings. Heat to the point of boiling. Diminish heat; stew, revealed, until potatoes and carrots are delicate, 9 minutes.

2. Include yellow squash and zucchini; cook until vegetables are delicate, 9 minutes longer. Serve or, whenever wanted, puree blend in clusters, including extra stock until wanted consistency is accomplished.

Salad Chard and White Bean Pasta

Total Time

Prep: 20 min. Cook: 20 min.

Makes

8 servings

Ingredients:

1 bundle (12 ounces) uncooked entire wheat or darker rice penne pasta

2 tablespoons olive oil

4 cups cut leeks (a white bit as it were)

1 cup cut sweet onion

4 garlic cloves, cut

1 tablespoon minced crisp savvy or 1 teaspoon scoured sage

1 enormous sweet potato, stripped and cut into 1/2-inch solid shapes

1 medium bundle Swiss chard (around 1 pound), cut into 1-inch cuts

1 can (15-1/2 ounces) extraordinary northern beans, flushed and depleted

3/4 teaspoon salt

1/4 teaspoon bean stew powder

1/4 teaspoon squashed red pepper drops 1/8 teaspoon ground nutmeg 1/8 teaspoon pepper

1/3 cup finely slashed crisp basil

1 tablespoon balsamic vinegar

2 cups marinara sauce, warmed

Directions:

1.   Cook pasta as indicated by bundle headings. Channel, holding 3/4 cup pasta water.

2.   In a 6-qt. stockpot, heat oil over medium warmth; saute leeks and onion until delicate, 5-7 minutes. Include garlic and sage; cook and mix 2 minutes.

3.   Include potato and chard; cook, secured, over medium-low warmth 5 minutes. Mix in beans, seasonings and held pasta water; cook, secured, until potato and chard are delicate, around 5 minutes.

4.   Include pasta, basil, and vinegar; hurl and warmth through. Present with sauce.

Cauliflower with Roasted Almond and Pepper Dip

Total Time

Prep: 40 min. Bake: 35 min.

Makes

10 servings (2-1/4 cups dip)

Ingredients:

10 cups water

1 cup olive oil, isolated

3/4 cup sherry or red wine vinegar, isolated

3 tablespoons salt

1 cove leaf

1 tablespoon squashed red pepper drops

1 enormous head cauliflower

1/2 cup entire almonds, toasted

1/2 cup delicate entire wheat or white bread morsels, toasted 1/2 cup fire-simmered squashed tomatoes

1 container (8 ounces) broiled sweet red peppers, depleted

2 tablespoons minced new parsley

2 garlic cloves

1 teaspoon sweet paprika

1/2 teaspoon salt

1/4 teaspoon newly ground pepper

Directions:

1.   In a 6-qt. stockpot, bring water, 1/2 cup oil, 1/2 cup sherry, salt, sound leaf, and pepper pieces to a bubble. Include cauliflower. Diminish heat; stew, revealed, until a blade effectively embeds into focus, 15-20 minutes, turning part of the way through cooking. Evacuate with an opened spoon; channel well on paper towels.

2.   Preheat broiler to 450°. Spot cauliflower on a lubed wire rack in a 15x10x1-in. heating dish. Prepare on a lower broiler rack until dim brilliant, 39 minutes.

3.   In the meantime, place almonds, bread morsels, tomatoes, cooked peppers, parsley, garlic, paprika, salt, and pepper in a nourishment processor; beat until finely cleaved. Include remaining sherry; process until mixed. Keep preparing while step by step including remaining oil in a constant flow. Present with cauliflower.

Spicy Grilled Broccoli

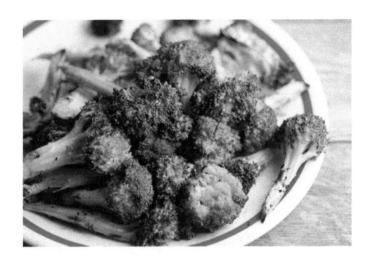

Total Time

Prep: 20 min. + standing Grill: 10 min.

Makes

6 servings

Ingredients:

2 packs broccoli

MARINADE:

1/2 cup olive oil

1/4 cup juice vinegar

1 teaspoon onion powder

1 teaspoon garlic powder

1 teaspoon smoked paprika

1/2 teaspoon salt

1/2 teaspoon squashed red pepper pieces 1/4 teaspoon pepper

Direction:

1.   Cut every broccoli pack into 6 pieces. In a 6-qt. stockpot, place a steamer container more than 1 in. of water. Spot broccoli in bushel. Heat water to the point of boiling. Decrease warmth to keep up a stew; steam, secured, 4-6 minutes or until fresh delicate.

2.   In an enormous bowl, whisk marinade fixings until mixed. Include broccoli; delicately hurl to cover. Let stand, secured, 15 minutes.

3.   Channel broccoli, saving marinade. Flame broil broccoli, secured, over medium warmth or cook 4 in. from heat 6-8 minutes or until broccoli is delicate, turning once. Whenever wanted, present withheld marinade.

Super-easy Chicken Noodle Soup

SmartPoints value: Green plan - 3SP, Blue plan - 2SP, Purple plan - 2SP

Total Time: 32 min, Prep time: 12 min, Cooking time: 20 min, Serves: 8

Nutritional value: Calories - 351.3, Carbs - 37.3g, Fat - 4.5g, Protein - 39.7g

In this recipe, I will make it easy for you to prepare a hearty soup for the whole family, all with just one pot. A big cup of 1 1/2 portion has only two SmartPoints value, so it's perfect for lunch, either to take to work or for your child's lunchbox, too.

Unlike other recipes like it, this one will be ready in just 32 minutes, not hours!

Now, pick up some ZeroPoint chicken breasts, frozen vegetables, a box of pasta, chicken broth, and a few more bits and pieces, and let's get you started on this family delight.

Ingredients

Black pepper - ¼ tsp

Chicken breast(s) (cooked) - 6 oz, chopped (skinless, boneless)

Salted butter - 2 tsp

Onion(s) (uncooked)- 1 large, well chopped

Table salt - 1½ tsp, divided

Chicken broth (reduced-sodium) - 64 oz

Pasta (uncooked) - 4 oz, small shape such as ditalini (about 1 cup)

Mixed vegetables (frozen) - 10 oz, such as peas, green beans, and carrots

Tomatoes (canned) - 15 oz, petite cut, rinsed and drained

Parmesan cheese (grated) - 1 Tbsp

Lemon juice (fresh) - 2 tsp

Fresh chives - ¼ cup(s), chopped (optional)

Instructions

1.   Melt two teaspoons of butter in a large stockpot over medium-low heat.

2.   Add well-chopped onion and 1/2 teaspoon of salt, then cook, often stirring, until the onion is soft and translucent; about 10 minutes.

3.   Add the broth in the chicken and increase the heat to high, then bring it to a boil.

4.   Put in the pasta, frozen vegetables, and tomatoes, then cook until pasta is soft; about 7 minutes.

5.   Stir in the chicken, lemon juice, cheese, remaining one teaspoon of salt, black pepper, and chives, then cook one more minute to heat through.

Hearty Ginger Soup

Serving: 4

Prep Time: 5 minutes

Cook Time: 5 minutes

Ingredients:

3 cups coconut almond milk

2 cups water

½ pound boneless chicken breast halves, cut into chunks 3 tablespoons fresh ginger root, minced 2 tablespoons fish sauce

¼ cup fresh lime juice

2 tablespoons green onions, sliced

1 tablespoon fresh cilantro, chopped

How To:

1.   Take a saucepan and add coconut almond milk and water.

2.   Bring the mixture to a boil and add the chicken strips.

3.   Reduce the warmth to medium and simmer for 3 minutes.

4.   Stir within the ginger, juice , and fish sauce.

5.   Sprinkle a couple of green onions and cilantro.

6.   Serve!

Nutrition (Per Serving)

Calories: 415

Fat: 39g

Carbohydrates: 8g

Protein: 14g

Tasty Tofu and Mushroom Soup

Serving: 8

Prep Time: 10 minutes

Cook Time: 10 minutes

Ingredients:

3 cups prepared dashi stock

¼ cup shiitake mushrooms, sliced

1 tablespoon miso paste

1 tablespoon coconut aminos

1/8 cup cubed soft tofu

1 green onion, diced

How To:

1.   Take a saucepan and add stock, bring back a boil.

2.   Add mushrooms, cook for 4 minutes.

3.   Take a bowl and add coconut aminos, miso paste and blend well.

4.   Pour the mixture into stock and let it cook for six minutes on simmer.

5.   Add diced green onions and enjoy!

Nutrition (Per Serving)

Calories: 100

Fat: 4g

Carbohydrates: 5g

Protein: 11

Ingenious Eggplant Soup

Serving: 8

Prep Time: 20 minutes

Cook Time: 15 minutes

Ingredients:

1 large eggplant, washed and cubed

1 tomato, seeded and chopped

1 small onion, diced

2 tablespoons parsley, chopped

2 tablespoons extra virgin olive oil

2 tablespoons distilled white vinegar

½ cup parmesan cheese, crumbled Sunflower seeds as needed

How To:

1.   Pre-heat your outdoor grill to medium-high.

2.   Pierce the eggplant a couple of times employing a knife/fork.

3.   Cook the eggplants on your grill for about quarter-hour until they're charred.

4.   forgot and permit them to chill .

5.   Remove the skin from the eggplant and dice the pulp.

6.   Transfer the pulp to a bowl and add parsley, onion, tomato, olive oil, feta cheese and vinegar.

7.   Mix well and chill for 1 hour.

8.   Season with sunflower seeds and enjoy!

Nutrition (Per Serving)

Calories: 99

Fat: 7g

Carbohydrates: 7g

Protein:3.4g

Loving Cauliflower Soup

Serving: 6

Prep Time: 10 minutes

Cook Time: 10 minutes

Ingredients:

4 cups vegetable stock

1-pound cauliflower, trimmed and chopped

7 ounces Kite ricotta/cashew cheese

4 ounces almond butter

Sunflower seeds and pepper to taste

How To:

1.   Take a skillet and place it over medium heat.

2.   Add almond butter and melt.

3.   Add cauliflower and sauté for two minutes.

4.   Add stock and convey mix to a boil.

5.   Cook until cauliflower is hard .

6.   Stir in cheese, sunflower seeds and pepper.

7.   Puree the combination using an immersion blender.

8.   Serve and enjoy!

Nutrition (Per Serving)

Calories: 143

Fat: 16g

Carbohydrates: 6g

Protein: 3.4g

Grilled Cod Fillets with Lemon Dill Butter

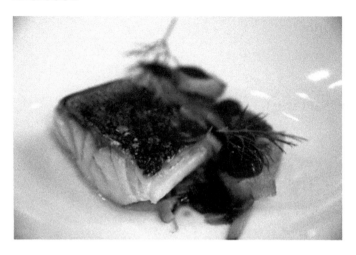

SmartPoints value: Green plan - 3SP, Blue plan - 2SP, Purple plan - 2SP

Total Time: 25 min, Prep time: 15 min, Cooking time: 10 min, Serves: 4

Nutritional value: Calories - 318.7g, Carbs - 6.7g, Fat - 13.0g, Protein - 41.7g

Grill the fish on slices of lemon topped with dill to add a delicious flavor to this dish. Become confident at grilling fish. With the layer of lemon slices, you can easily prevent the fish from sticking to the grate. To make use of a stovetop, prepare a grill pan by preheating it over medium-high heat until it is almost smoking, then continue with the recipe. The mixture of lemon, butter, and dill creates a robust sauce that becomes ready in minutes, even though it tastes like you spent hours preparing it. It is preferable to serve this dish with grilled asparagus.

Ingredients

Olive oil -2 tsp

Uncooked Atlantic cod - 24 oz, or another firm white fish like tilapia (four 6-oz fillets)

Table salt - ½ tsp

Lemon(s) (sliced 1/4-in thick) - 2 medium (you'll need 12 slices total)

Dill - 2 tsp, chopped

Dill - 4 sprig(s)

Light butter - 4 tsp (at room temp.)

Lemon zest - 1 tsp

Instructions

1.   Get your grill ready by preheating to medium-high heat. Continue the heating for at least 10 minutes after it reaches the

desired temperature, then scrape the grate clean with a steel brush and coat it lightly with oil.

2. While the grill heats up, pat the fish dry and sprinkle salt on it.

3. Place three lemon slices on the grill carefully, overlapping slightly, and top it with a dill sprig and fish fillet.

4. Repeat the same with the remaining lemon, dill, and fish. Cover the grill and cook without turning for 8-10 minutes until the fish is opaque all the way through and yields easily to a thin-bladed knife.

5. While the cooking is on-going, mix the butter, chopped dill, and zest in a small shallow bowl.

6. Transfer each lemon-dill-fish portion to a plate using two thin-bladed spatulas and top them with 1 1/2 tsp of lemon-dill butter and serve (serving the lemon slices is optional).

Spicy Baked Shrimp

Serving: 4

Prep Time: 10 minutes

Cook Time: 25 minutes + 2-4 hours

Ingredients:

½ ounce large shrimp, peeled and deveined Cooking spray as needed

1 teaspoon low sodium coconut amines

1 teaspoon parsley

½ teaspoon olive oil

½ tablespoon honey

1 tablespoon lemon juice

How To:

1.   Pre-heat your oven to 450 degrees F.

2.   Take a baking dish and grease it well.

3.   Mix altogether the ingredients and toss.

4.   Transfer to oven and bake for 8 minutes until shrimp turns pink.

5.   Serve and enjoy!

Nutrition (Per Serving)

Calories: 321

Fat: 9g

Carbohydrates: 44g

Protein: 22g

Shrimp and Cilantro Meal

Serving: 4

Prep Time: 10 minutes

Cook Time: 5 minutes

Ingredients:

¾ pounds shrimp, deveined and peeled

tablespoons fresh lime juice

¼ teaspoon cloves, minced

½ teaspoon ground cumin

1 tablespoon olive oil

1 ¼ cups fresh cilantro, chopped

1 teaspoon lime zest

½ teaspoon sunflower seeds

¼ teaspoon pepper

Direction

1. Take an outsized sized bowl and add shrimp, cumin, garlic, juice, ginger and toss well.

2. Take an outsized sized non-stick skillet and add oil, allow the oil to heat up over medium-high heat.

3. Add shrimp mixture and sauté for 4 minutes.

4. Remove the warmth and add cilantro, lime zest, sunflower seeds, and pepper.

5. Mix well and serve hot!

Nutrition (Per Serving)

Calories: 177

Fat: 6g

Carbohydrates: 2g

Protein: 27g

The Original Dijon Fish

Serving: 2

Prep Time: 3 minutes

Cook Time: 12 minutes

Ingredients:

1 perch, flounder or sole fish florets

1 tablespoon Dijon mustard

1 ½ teaspoons lemon juice

teaspoon low sodium Worcestershire sauce, low sodium
tablespoons Italian seasoned bread crumbs 1 almond butter
flavored cooking spray

How To:

1.   Preheat your oven to 450 degrees F.

2.   Take an 11 x 7-inch baking dish and arrange your fillets
carefully.

3.   Take a little sized bowl and add juice, Worcester sauce,
mustard and blend it well.

4. Pour the combination over your fillet.

5. Sprinkle an honest amount of breadcrumbs.

6. Bake for 12 minutes until fish flakes off easily.

7. Cut the fillet in half portions and enjoy!

Nutrition (Per Serving)

Calories: 125

Fat: 2g

Carbohydrates: 6g

Protein: 21g

Lemony Garlic Shrimp

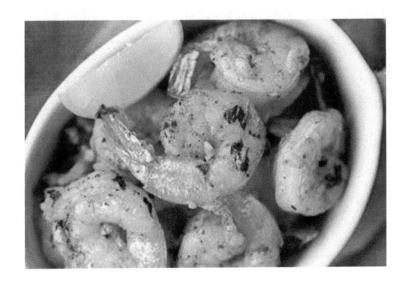

Serving: 4

Prep Time: 5-10 minutes

Cook Time: 10-15 minutes

Ingredients:

1 ¼ pounds shrimp, boiled or steamed

tablespoons garlic, minced

¼ cup lemon juice

tablespoons olive oil

¼ cup parsley

How To:

1.   Take alittle skillet and place over medium heat, add garlic and oil and stir-cook for 1 minute.

2.   Add parsley, juice and season with sunflower seeds and pepper accordingly.

3.   Add shrimp during a large bowl and transfer the mixture from the skillet over the shrimp.

4.   Chill and serve.

5.   Enjoy!

Nutrition (Per Serving)

Calories: 130

Fat: 3g

Carbohydrates:2g

Protein:22g

Chicken Tortilla Soup

SmartPoints value: Green plan - 4SP, Blue plan - 2SP, Purple plan - 2SP

Total Time: 45 min, Prep time: 15 min, Cooking time: 30 min, Serves: 6

Nutritional value:

Calories - 200, Carbs - 24g, Fat - 9g, Protein - 7g

Preparing this soup is very easy. Once you have chopped and sautéed the vegetables, the rest of the cooking is practically hands-off. You will simmer the chicken in a flavored broth made with fire-roasted tomatoes and lime juice. Doing this will give you some extra minutes to put together a quick salad or other simple side dishes. Chicken breasts (boneless, skinless) work well in this soup, but you can use chicken thighs as well. If you'd like to make things more interesting, don't de-seed the jalapeño completely.

Ingredients

Cilantro (chopped) - 1 cup(s)

Chili powder - 1 tsp

Chicken broth (reduced-sodium) - 6 cup(s)

Olive oil - 1 tsp

Uncooked onion(s) (chopped) - 1½ cup(s)

Kosher salt -1½ tsp

Minced Garlic - 4 tsp

Jalapeño pepper(s) - 1 medium (seeded and minced)

Tomatoes (canned, diced)- 15 oz, fire roasted-variety, drained

Uncooked chicken breast - 20 oz (boneless, skinless)

Lime juice (fresh) - ⅓ cup(s)

Mexican-style cheese (Shredded reduced) - 6 Tbsp

Tortilla chips (crushed) - 12 chip(s)

Instructions

1.   Set a soup pot over medium heat and preheat.

2.   Toss in the chopped onion and salt, then cook, often stirring, until the onion gets soft; 5-10 minutes.

3.   Add garlic, chili powder, and jalapeno, then cook for one minute.

4.   Put in your broth, tomatoes, lime juice, and chicken, then stir to combine.

5. Simmer and cook until the chicken breasts cook through; about 20 minutes.

6. Remove the chicken breasts from the soup and shred them with two forks, then return the shredded chicken to the pot with cilantro.

7. Serve your soup garnished with tortilla chips and cheese.

Chicken Piccata Stir-Fry

SmartPoints value: Green plan - 4SP, Blue plan - 2SP, Purple plan - 2SP

Total Time: 25 min, Prep time: 20 min, Cooking time: 5 min, Serves: 4

Nutritional value: Cal - 190.5, Carbs - 5.6g, Fat - 9.4g, Protein - 18.6g

This dish is a combination of the classic Italian chicken piccata and Asian stir-fry.

Ingredients

Black pepper (freshly ground) - ¼ tsp

Capers (rinsed)- 1 Tbsp

Chicken broth (fat-free) - ½ cup(s)

Cornstarch (divided) - 2 tsp

Dry sherry (divided)- 3 Tbsp

Table salt (divided) - ¾ tsp

Soy sauce (low sodium) - 1 Tbsp

Peanut oil (divided) - 4 tsp, or vegetable oil

Uncooked chicken breast (boneless, skinless) - 1 pound(s), cut into quarter-inch-thick slices

Uncooked shallot(s) - 1 medium, thinly sliced Minced Garlic - 1 Tbsp

String beans (uncooked) - 2 cup(s), cut into two-inch lengths Parsley (fresh, chopped) - 2 Tbsp

Lemon(s) - ½ medium, cut into four

Instructions

1.   Prepare a clean medium-sized bowl and mix chicken, 1 tsp of cornstarch,1 Tbsp of dry sherry,1/2 tsp salt, and pepper in it.

2.   Next, get a small bowl and combine broth, soy sauce, remaining 2 Tbsp of dry sherry, and 1 tsp of cornstarch.

3.   Preheat a fourteen-inch flat-bottomed wok or twelve-inch skillet over high heat to the point where a drop of water will evaporate within 1 to 2 seconds of contact, then swirl in one Tbsp oil.

4.   Add shallots and garlic, then stir-fry for 10 seconds. Push the shallot mixture to the sides of the wok and add the chicken, then spread in one layer in the wok.

5. Cook the chicken undisturbed for 60 seconds, allowing the chicken to begin searing, then stir-fry another 60 seconds until chicken is no longer pink but not yet thoroughly cooked.

6. Swirl the chicken in the remaining 1 tsp oil and toss in green beans and capers. Sprinkle on the remaining 1/4 tsp of salt and stir-fry for 30 seconds or until just combined.

7. Swirl the chicken in the broth mixture and stir-fry for 1-2 minutes or until the chicken is cooked through, with the sauce slightly thickened.

8. Sprinkle the parsley on it and serve with lemon wedges.

Ranch Meatballs

SmartPoints value: Green plan - 4SP, Blue plan - 4SP, Purple plan – 5SP

Total Time: 20mins, Prep time: 10 mins, Cooking time: 30mins, Serves: 4

Nutritional value: Calories - 195, Carbs - 6g, Fat - 6g, Protein - 26g

Meatball recipes are delicious protein recipes that are so satisfying and tasty. They can be a fun and easy meal. It becomes easier to prepare the perfect sized meatballs using a meatball shaper.

Ingredients

Ground beef (96/4) (extra lean) - 1 lb

Panko breadcrumbs - 1/3 cup(s)

Egg substitute (Liquid, like egg beaters) - 1/4 cup

Olive oil - 1 tsp

Onion powder - 1 tbsp

Garlic powder - 1 tbsp

Dill (dried) - 2 tsp

Parsley (dried) - 2 tsp

Basil (dried) - 2 tsp

Salt and pepper - Add to taste

Instructions

1.   Combine all the ingredients by hand in a large bowl and shape it into about 24 meatballs.

2.   Apply heat to the oil in a large non-stick skillet over medium-high heat.

3.   Place meatballs in the pan and cook for about 1-2 minutes on each side, until all sides get lightly browned.

4.   Reduce the heat to medium-low and pour in half a cup of water. Cover it and cook, occasionally stirring, until meatballs cook thoroughly; about 10-12 minutes.

Note: Meatballs are a perfect simple Weight Watchers dinner recipe for those who are watching Points but also savour the flavour

Beef Orzo with Feta

SmartPoints value: Green plan - 8SP, Blue plan - 8SP, Purple plan – 8SP

Total Time: 35mins, Prep time: 10mins, Cooking time: 25mins, Serves: 6

Nutritional value: Calories - 325, Carbs – 44g, Fat – 5.5g, Protein – 25g

Beef Orzo is one of those types of meals that you'll love to prepare now and then. The instructions for preparation are quite easy to follow, and the meal is just delicious. If you haven't tried it, you are missing out big time. You should give it a try for your next family dinner or friends gathering. This most satisfying weight-watching dinner recipe is perfect for warming you and your family up on a chilly fall evening.

Ingredients

Ground beef (extra-lean) - 1 lb

Whole wheat orzo - 10 oz

Onion (finely chopped) - 1 large

Garlic (minced) - 4 cloves

Cinnamon (ground) - 1 tsp

Oregano (dried) - 2 tsp

Can tomatoes (crushed) - One 26oz

Reduced-fat feta cheese (crumbled) - 1/3 cup

Salt & pepper - Add to taste

Instructions

1.   Prepare whole orzo wheat according to package directions. Drain it and set aside.

2.   While the wheat is cooking, spray a large skillet with nonfat cooking spray, and set it over medium-high heat. Toss in some beef and cook until it mostly cooks through.

3.   Put in onions, oregano, garlic, cinnamon, salt, and pepper. Sauté the dish until the onions are tender and the beef cooks all the way through.

4.   Pour the crushed tomatoes into the skillet with the beef mixture, and cook on medium heat. Continue to cook, while occasionally stirring, until the mixture thickens; about 15 minutes.

5.   Dish the beef sauce with orzo and place in serving bowls. Top each bowl with 1 tbsp of feta.

Gentle Blackberry Crumble

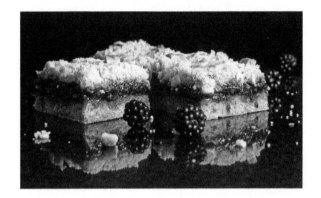

Serving: 4

Prep Time: 10 minutes

Cook Time: 45 minutes

Smart Points: 4

Ingredients:

½ cup coconut flour

½ cup banana, peeled and mashed

6 tablespoons water

3 cups fresh blackberries

½ cup arrowroot flour

1 ½ teaspoons baking soda

4 tablespoons almond butter, melted

1 tablespoon fresh lemon juice

How To:

1. Pre-heat your oven to 300 degrees F.

2. Take a baking dish and grease it lightly.

3. Take a bowl and mix all of the ingredients except the blackberries, mix well.

4. Place blackberries in the bottom of your baking dish and top with flour.

5. Bake for 40 minutes.

6. Serve and enjoy!

Nutrition (Per Serving)

Calories: 12

Fat: 7g

Carbohydrates: 10g

Protein: 4g

Mini Minty Happiness

Serving: 12

Prep Time: 45 minutes

Cooking Time: None Freeze Time: 2 hours

Ingredients:

2 teaspoons vanilla extract

1 ½ cups coconut oil

1 ¼ cups sunflower seed almond butter ½ cup dried parsley

1 teaspoon peppermint extract

A pinch of sunflower seeds

1 cup dark chocolate chips Stevia to taste

How To:

1.   Melt together coconut oil and dark chocolate chips over a double boiler.

2.   Take a food processor, add all the ingredients into it and pulse until smooth.

3. Pour into round molds.

4. Let it freeze.

Nutrition (Per Serving)

Total Carbs: 7g

Fiber: 1g

Protein: 3g

Fat: 25g

Astonishing Maple Pecan Bacon Slices

Serving: 12

Prep Time: 10 minutes

Cooking Time: 25 minutes

Freeze Time: None

Ingredients:

tablespoon sugar-free maple syrup

12 bacon slices

Granulated Stevia to taste

15-20 drops Stevia For the coating:

4 tablespoons dark cocoa powder

¼ cup pecans, chopped

15-20 drops Stevia

How To:

1.   Take a baking tray and lay the bacon slices on it.

2.   Rub with maple syrup and Stevia, flip the slices and do the same with the other side.

3.   Bake for 10-15 minutes at 227 degrees F.

4.   After they've baked, drain the bacon grease.

5.   To form a batter, mix the bacon grease, Stevia and cocoa powder.

6.   Dip the bacon slices into the batter and roll in the chopped pecans.

7.   Allow to air dry until the chocolate hardens.

Nutrition (Per Serving)

Total Carbs: 1g

Fiber: 0g

Protein: 10g

Fat: 11g

Generous Maple and Pecan Bites

Serving: 12

Prep Time: 10 minutes

Cooking Time: 25 minutes

Freeze Time: None

Ingredients:

1 cup almond meal

½ cup coconut oil

½ cup flaxseed meal

½ cup sugar-free chocolate chips

2 cups pecans, chopped

½ cup sugar-free maple syrup

20-25 drops Stevia

How To:

1.   Take a baking dish and spread the pecans.

2.   Bake at 350 degrees F until aromatic.

3.   This will usually take from 6 to 8 minutes.

4.   Meanwhile, sift together all the dry ingredients.

5.   Add the roasted pecans to the mix and mix them properly.

6.   Add the coconut oil and maple syrup.

7.   Stir to make a thick, sticky mixture.

8.   Take a bread pan lined with parchment paper, and pour the mixture into it.

9.   Bake for about 18 minutes.

10.   Slice and serve.

Nutrition (Per Serving)

Total Carbs: 6g

Fiber: 0g

Protein: 5g

Fat: 30g

Carrot Ball Delight

Serving: 4

Prep Time: 10 minutes

Cook Time: Nil

Ingredients:

6 Medjool dates pitted

1 carrot, finely grated

¼ cup raw walnuts

¼ cup unsweetened coconut, shredded

1 teaspoon nutmeg

1/8 teaspoon sunflower seeds

How To:

1.   Take a food processor and add dates, ¼ cup of grated carrots, sunflower seeds coconut, nutmeg.

2.   Mix well and puree the mixture.

3.   Add the walnuts and remaining ¼ cup of carrots.

4. Pulse the mixture until you have a chunky texture.

5. Form balls using your hand and roll them up in coconut.

6. Top with carrots and chill.

7. Enjoy!

Nutrition (Per Serving)

Calories: 326

Fat: 16g

Carbohydrates: 42g

Protein: 3g

Awesome Brownie Muffins

Serving: 5

Prep Time: 10 minutes

Cooking Time: 35 minutes

Ingredients:

1 cup golden flaxseed meal

¼ cup cocoa powder

1 tablespoon cinnamon

½ tablespoon baking powder

½ teaspoon sunflower seeds

1 whole large egg

2 tablespoons coconut oil

¼ cup sugar-free caramel syrup

½ cup pumpkin puree

1 teaspoon vanilla extract

1 teaspoon apple cider vinegar

¼ cup almonds, slivered

How To:

1.   Pre-heat your oven to 350 degrees F.

2.   Take a mixing bowl and add all of the listed ingredients and mix everything well.

3.   Take your desired number of muffin tins and line them with paper liners.

4.   Scoop the batter into the muffin tins, filling them to about 1/4 of the liner.

5.   Sprinkle a bit of almond on top.

6.   Place them in your oven and bake for 15 minutes.

7.   Serve warm.

Nutrition (Per Serving)

Total Carbs: 16

Fiber: 2g

Protein: 3g

Fat: 31g

Spice Friendly Muffins

Serving: 12

Prep Time: 5 minutes

Cooking Time: 45minute

Ingredients:

½ cup raw hemp hearts

½ cup flaxseeds

¼ cup chia seeds

2 tablespoons Psyllium husk powder

1 tablespoon cinnamon

Stevia taste

½ teaspoon baking powder

½ teaspoon sunflower seeds

1 cup of water

How To:

1.   Pre-heat your oven to 350 degrees F.

2.   Line muffin tray with liners.

3.   Take a large sized mixing bowl and add peanut almond butter, pumpkin, sweetener, coconut almond milk, flaxseed and mix well.

4.   Keep stirring until the mixture has been thoroughly combined.

5.   Take another bowl and add baking powder, spices and coconut flour.

6.   Mix well.

7.   Add the dry ingredients into the wet bowl and stir until the coconut flour has mixed well.

8.   Allow it to sit for a while until the coconut flour has absorbed all of the moisture.

9.   Divide the mixture amongst your muffin tins and bake for 45 minutes.

10.   Enjoy!

Nutrition (Per Serving)

Total Carbs: 7g

Fiber: 3g

Protein: 6g

Fat: 15g

Spicy Apple Crisp

Nutritional Facts

servings per container	5
Prep Total	**10 min**
Serving Size	7
Amount per serving **Calories**	**0.2%**
	% Daily Value
Total Fat 8g	**22%**
Saturated Fat 1g	51%
Trans Fat 0g	2%
Cholesterol	**2%**
Sodium 20mg	**0.2%**
Total Carbohydrate 70g	**540%**
Dietary Fiber 3g	1%
Total Sugar 6g	1%
Protein 6g	24
Vitamin C 4mcg	170%
Calcium 160mg	12%
Iron 2mg	210%
Potassium 30mg	21%

Ingredients:

8 cooking apples

4 oz or 150 g flour

7 oz or 350 g brown sugar

5 oz or 175 g vegan butter

¼ tablespoon ground cinnamon

¼ tablespoon ground nutmeg

Zest of one lemon

1 tablespoon fresh lemon juice

Instructions:

Peel, quarter and core cooking apples.

Cut apple quarters into thin slices and place them in a bowl.

Blend nutmeg and cinnamon then sprinkle over apples.

Sprinkle with lemon rind.

Add lemon juice and toss to blend.

Arrange slices in a large baking dish.

Make a mixture of sugar, flour, and vegan butter in a mixing bowl then put over apples, smoothing it over.

Place the dish in the oven.

Bake at 370°F, 190°C or gas mark 5 for 60 minutes, until browned and apples are tender.

Apple Cake

Nutritional Facts

servings per container	8
Prep Total	**10 min**
Serving Size	2
Amount per serving **Calories**	**0%**
	% Daily Value
Total Fat 4g	**210%**
Saturated Fat 3g	32%
Trans Fat 2g	2%
Cholesterol	**8%**
Sodium 300mg	**0.2%**
Total Carbohydrate 20g	**50%**
Dietary Fiber 1g	1%
Total Sugar 1g	1%
Protein 3g	
Vitamin C 1mcg	18%
Calcium 20mg	1%
Iron 8mg	12%
Potassium 70mg	21%

Ingredients:

2 oz or 50 g flour

3 tablespoon baking powder

½ tablespoon of salt

2 tablespoon vegan shortening

¼ pint or 125 ml unsweetened soya milk 4 or 5 apples

4 oz or 110 g sugar

1 tablespoon cinnamon

Instructions:

Sift together flour, baking powder, and salt.

Add shortening and rub in very lightly.

Add milk slowly to make soft dough and mix.

Place on floured board and roll out ½ inch or 1 cm thick.

Put into shallow greased pan.

Wash, pare, core, \ and cut apples into sections; press them into a dough.

Sprinkle with sugar and dust with cinnamon.

Bake at 375°F, 190°C, or gas mark 5 for 30 minutes or until apples are tender and brown.

Serve with soya cream.

Apple Charlotte

Nutritional Facts

servings per container	5
Prep Total	**10 min**
Serving Size	4
Amount per serving **Calories**	**60%**
	% Daily Value
Total Fat 1g	**200%**
Saturated Fat 20g	3%
Trans Fat 14g	2%
Cholesterol	**2%**
Sodium 210mg	**2%**
Total Carbohydrate 7g	**210%**
Dietary Fiber 1g	9%
Total Sugar 21g	8%
Protein 4g	
Vitamin C 4mcg	22%
Calcium 30mg	17%
Iron 8mg	110%
Potassium 12mg	2%

Ingredients:

2 lbs or 900 g good cooking apples

4 oz or 50 g almonds (chopped)

2 oz or 50 g currants and sultanas mixed

1 stick cinnamon (about 3 inches or 7 cm long)

Juice of ½ a lemon

Whole bread (cut very thinly) spread

Sugar to taste.

Instructions:

1.   Pare, core, and cut up the apples.

2.   Stew the apples with a teacupful of water and the cinnamon, until the apples have become a pulp.

3.   Remove the cinnamon, and add sugar, lemon juice, the almonds, and the currants and sultanas (previously picked, washed, and dried).

4.   Mix all well and allow the mixture to cool.

5.   Grease a pie-dish and line it with thin slices of bread and butter,

6.   Then place on it a layer of apple mixture, repeat the layers, finishing with slices of bread and vegan butter.

7.   Bake at 375°F, 190°C or gas mark 5 for 45 minutes.

Mixed Berries Smoothie

Serving: 2

Prep Time: 4 minutes

Cook Time: 0 minutes

Ingredients:

¼ cup frozen blueberries

¼ cup frozen blackberries

1 cup unsweetened almond milk

1 teaspoon vanilla bean extract

3 teaspoons flaxseeds

1 scoop chilled Greek yogurt

Stevia as needed

How To:

1.   Mix everything in a blender and emulsify.

2.   Pulse the mixture four time until you have your desired thickness.

3.   Pour the mixture into a glass and enjoy!

Nutrition (Per Serving)

Calories: 221

Fat: 9g

Protein: 21g

Carbohydrates: 10g

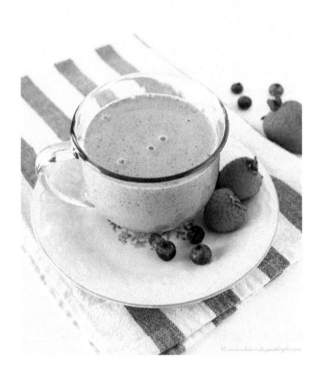

Satisfying Berry and Almond Smoothie

Serving: 4

Prep Time: 10 minutes

Cook Time: nil

Ingredients:

1 cup blueberries, frozen

1 whole banana

½ cup almond milk

1 tablespoon almond butter

Water as needed

How To:

1.   Add the listed ingredients to your blender and blend well until you have a smoothie-like texture.

2.   Chill and serve.

3.   Enjoy!

Nutrition (Per Serving)

Calories: 321

Fat: 11g

Carbohydrates: 55g

Protein: 5g

Simple Rice Mushroom Risotto

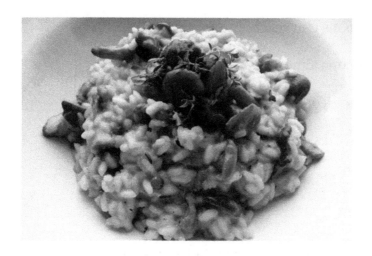

Serving: 4

Prep Time: 5 minutes

Cook Time: 15 minutes

Ingredients:

4 ½ cups cauliflower, riced

3 tablespoons coconut oil

1-pound Portobello mushrooms, thinly sliced

1-pound white mushrooms, thinly sliced

2 shallots, diced

¼ cup organic vegetable broth

Sunflower seeds and pepper to taste

3 tablespoons chives, chopped

4 tablespoons almond butter

½ cup kite ricotta/cashew cheese, grated

How To:

1.   Use a food processor and pulse cauliflower florets until riced.

2.   Take a large saucepan and heat up 2 tablespoons oil over medium-high flame.

3.   Add mushrooms and sauté for 3 minutes until mushrooms are tender.

4.   Clear saucepan of mushrooms and liquid and keep them on the side.

5.   Add the rest of the 1 tablespoon oil to skillet.

6.   Toss shallots and cook for 60 seconds.

7.   Add cauliflower rice, stir for 2 minutes until coated with oil.

8. Add broth to riced cauliflower and stir for 5 minutes.

9. Remove pot from heat and mix in mushrooms and liquid.

10. Add chives, almond butter, parmesan cheese.

11. Season with sunflower seeds and pepper.

12. Serve and enjoy!

Nutrition (Per Serving)

Calories: 438

Fat: 17g

Carbohydrates: 15g

Protein: 12g

Hearty Green Bean Roast

Serving: 4

Prep Time: 10 minutes

Cook Time: 20 minutes

Ingredients:

1 whole egg

2 tablespoons olive oil

Sunflower seeds and pepper to taste

1-pound fresh green beans

5 ½ tablespoons grated parmesan cheese

How To:

1.   Pre-heat your oven to 400 degrees F.

2.   Take a bowl and whisk in eggs with oil and spices.

3.   Add beans and mix well.

4.   Stir in parmesan cheese and pour the mix into baking pan (lined with parchment paper).

5.   Bake for 15-20 minutes.

6.   Serve warm and enjoy!

Nutrition (Per Serving)

Calories: 216

Fat: 21g

Carbohydrates: 7g

Protein: 9g

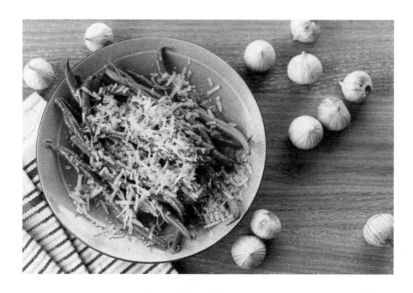

Almond and Blistered Beans

Serving: 4

Prep Time: 10 minutes

Cook Time: 20 minutes

Ingredients:

1-pound fresh green beans, ends trimmed

1 ½ tablespoon olive oil

¼ teaspoon sunflower seeds

1 ½ tablespoons fresh dill, minced

Juice of 1 lemon

¼ cup crushed almonds

Sunflower seeds as needed

How To:

1.   Pre-heat your oven to 400 degrees F.

2.   Add the green beans with your olive oil and also the sunflower seeds.

3.   Then spread them in one single layer on a large sized sheet pan.

4.   Roast it for 10 minutes and stir, then roast for another 8-10 minutes.

5.   Remove from the oven and keep stirring in the lemon juice alongside the dill.

6.   Top it with crushed almonds and some flaked sunflower seeds and serve.

Nutrition (Per Serving)

Calories: 347

Fat: 16g

Carbohydrates: 6g

Protein: 45g

Tomato Platter

Serving: 8

Prep Time: 10 minutes + Chill time

Cook Time: Nil

Ingredients:

1/3 cup olive oil

1 teaspoon sunflower seeds

2 tablespoons onion, chopped

¼ teaspoon pepper

½ a garlic, minced

1 tablespoon fresh parsley, minced

3 large fresh tomatoes, sliced

1 teaspoon dried basil

¼ cup red wine vinegar

How To:

1.   Take a shallow dish and arrange tomatoes in the dish.

2.   Add the rest of the ingredients in a mason jar, cover the jar and shake it well.

3.   Pour the mix over tomato slices.

4.   Let it chill for 2-3 hours.

5.   Serve!

Nutrition (Per Serving)

Calories: 350

Fat: 28g

Carbohydrates: 10g

Protein: 14g

Lightning Source UK Ltd.
Milton Keynes UK
UKHW050441230421
382423UK00004B/56